Cancer

Of

Vital Organs Of The Body

Causes And Prevention

By

Wilfred Hastings

Disclaimer

Copyright © by **Professor Wilfred Hastings** 2022. All rights reserved.Before this document is duplicated or reproduced in any manner, the publisher's consent must be gained. Therefore, the contents within can neither be stored electronically, transferred, nor kept in a database. Neither in Part nor full can the document be copied, scanned, faxed, or retained without approval from the publisher or creator.

Table Of Contents

Causes Of Liver Cancer

Prevention Of Liver Cancer

Introduction

Understanding the importance of cancer prevention in today's environment is essential for general wellbeing. This book details certain cancer illness causes and preventions. A better, cancer-free life can be attained by raising awareness of certain illnesses and putting a priority on preventative measures. The fight against cancer requires constant health checks, a healthy lifestyle, and getting medical help for any unsettling signs. Keep in mind that prevention and early detection are crucial for better outcomes and a higher quality of life. Stay vigilant and healthy.

What Is Cancer?

Cancer is a sickness where a portion of the body's cells develop wildly and spread to different parts of the body.

Cancer growth can begin at any place in the human body, which is composed of trillions of cells. Regularly, human cells develop and increase (through an process called cell division) to frame new cells as the body needs them. At the point when cells become old or become harmed, they die, and new cells have their spot.

Now and again this systematic interaction separates, and unusual or harmed cells develop and duplicate when they shouldn't. These cells might shape cancers, which are pieces of tissue. Growths can be destructive or not carcinogenic (harmless).

Destructive growths spread into, or attack, close to tissues and can venture out to far-off places in the body to shape new cancers (a cycle called metastasis). Dangerous cancers may likewise be called harmful growths. Numerous malignant growths structure strong growths, yet tumors of the blood, like leukemias, for the most part, don't.

Harmless growths don't spread into, or attack, close to tissues. At the point when taken out, harmless growths generally don't bounce back, while carcinogenic cancers some of the time do. Harmless growths can at times be very huge, in any case. Some can cause serious side effects or be dangerous, like harmless growths in the mind

Breast Cancer

What is breast cancer?

Breast cancer begins in your bosom tissue. It happens when breast cells transform (change) and outgrow control, making a mass of tissue (growth). Like different tumors,these cells can attack and develop into the tissue encompassing your bosom. It can likewise go to different places of your body and structure new growths. At that point when this occurs, it's called metastasis.

What causes breast cancer?

Breast cancer occur when unusual cells in your bosom partition and duplicate. Yet, specialists don't know precisely the exact thing that causes this cycle to start in any case.

In some cases, research demonstrates that there are a few factors that might build your possibilities for creating breast cancer. These include:

Sex. Ladies are significantly more prone to foster bosom malignant growth than men.

Family ancestry and hereditary qualities. Assuming you have guardians, kin, kids or other direct relations who've been determined to have bosom malignant growth, you're bound to foster the sickness eventually in your life. Around 5% to 10% of breast cancer growths are because of single unusual qualities that are passed down from guardians to kids, and that can be found by hereditary testing.

Smoking. Tobacco use has been connected to a wide range of sorts of cancer growth, including breat disease(cancer).

Corpulence. Having corpulence can expand your risk of breast cancer and bosom disease repeat.

Radiation openness. Assuming that you've had earlier radiation treatment — particularly to your head, neck or chest — you're bound to foster bosom disease.

Chemical substitution treatment. Individuals who use chemical substitution treatment (HRT) have a higher risk of being determined to have bosom disease.

There are numerous different elements that can build your possibilities for creating breast cancer. Converse with your medical care supplier to see whether you're in danger.

Side Effects Of Breasts Disease

Various individuals have various side effects of breasts cancer. Certain individuals have no signs or side effects by any means.

A few admonition indications of breasts cancer are —

Breast lymph, An abnormality in your chest Extending or bulges around your collarbone or armpits can be achieved by a bosom disease that has spread to lymph centers in those areas. The development can happen even before you can feel a bunch in your chest. If you have extended, make sure to permit your prosperity group to rapidly be aware.

Breast and Nipples pain.various things can cause areola trickiness or anguishing areolas. Close by pain or responsiveness, you can moreover experience shivering, redness or changes in the outer layer of your skin around your areola.

A significant part of the time, sore areolas are achieved by hormonal changes from pregnancy or female cycle, responsive qualities or grinding from clothing. In unprecedented cases, it will in general be a sign of a difficult sickness like chest dangerous development. Your clinical consideration provider should evaluate any exacerbation that is joined by delivery or anomalies at the earliest open door.

Everyone experiences areola aggravation or delicacy surprisingly.

Few Different Ways Of Forestalling Breast Cancer

- Avoid weight gain (obesity).
- Carve out opportunity to keep away from pressure through work out(exercise).
- Don't smoke
- **IV.**Eat Your Natural items and Vegetables - and Limit Alcohol
- If you're having any disturbance or pain in your chest or breast region do well to notify your health team about it or see a doctor.

Kidneys Cancer

Kidney sickness or cancer occurs when weird cells in both of the kidneys start to separate and fill in an uncontrolled way.

Side effects

Kidney cancer often shows no symptoms or indicators in its early stages. Several signs could develop gradually over time, including:

- Your urine may contain blood and be pink, crimson, or cola-colored.

- Your back or side pain is persistent.
- Diminished appetite
- Unreported decrease of weight
- Tiredness
- Fever

Causes Of Kidneys Cancer

Despite the precise origin of kidney cancer is unknown, there exist certain warning signs that might increase your risk of contracting the disease. These consist of:

<u>Smoking</u>: Smokers have a higher risk of developing kidney cancer. The longer a person smokes, the greater the risk is as well.

<u>Obesity</u>: increases the risk of kidney cancer. Generally speaking, a person's risk rises as their weight does.

A increased risk of kidney cancer has been linked to high blood pressure, or hypertension.

<u>Family history</u>: People who have a history of kidney cancer

may be more susceptible to developing the disease themselves.

<u>Radiation therapy</u>: Women who have undergone radiation therapy for cancer of the reproductive organs may have a slightly increased chance of developing kidney cancer.

Easy Steps To Prevent Kidney Cancer

By following these preventive steps, you can significantly reduce your risk of developing kidney cancer, a serious condition that affects millions of people worldwide.

I.A Healthy Diet: Eating a balanced, nutrient-rich diet is crucial for preventing kidney cancer. A variety of fruits, vegetables, whole grains, and lean meats should be present in each of your daily meals. Limit your intake of sodium, unhealthy fats, and processed meals. Additionally, drinking lots of water can have a huge positive impact on your kidneys.

II.Quit smoking: A substantial risk factor for kidney cancer is smoking. Your kidneys can sustain damage and lose functionality due to the dangerous compounds found in cigarettes. Quitting smoking lowers your risk
of kidney cancer development and enhances general health. To successfully stop smoking, get

help from a professional or join a support group.

III. Finance A Healthy Weight: Kidney cancer is one of many malignancies that obesity makes more likely. Your risk of contracting this illness can be decreased by keeping a healthy weight. To keep your weight within a healthy range, get frequent exercise by walking, running, or swimming. Determine the best fitness program for your health situation by speaking with your doctor.

IV. Reduce Exposure To Harmful Chemical:In order to avoid kidney cancer, dangerous material exposure must be minimized. Reduce your exposure to industrial chemicals, pesticides, and certain solvents that can harm your kidneys. Make sure the proper safety precautions are in place if you work in such settings. Limit your alcohol intake, and stay away from narcotics, which can also damage your kidneys.

V. Health Check-up Regularly:You must monitor your general health, particularly the health of your kidneys, with regular medical exams. The early detection of any potential problems is made possible by these

examinations. Consult with your healthcare practitioner about the precise exams that can evaluate your kidney health and look for any indications of kidney cancer. Treatment results are greatly enhanced by early discovery.

Lungs Cancer

Unchecked cell division in your lungs is the main cause of lung cancer. As part of their typical operation, your cells divide and create new duplicates of themselves. However, occasionally they experience modifications (mutations) that lead them to continue producing more of themselves when they shouldn't. Damaged cells dividing uncontrollably create masses, or tumors, of tissue that eventually keep your organs from working properly.

A person develops lung cancer when aberrant cells begin to proliferate out of control. The lungs' inability to function properly and the potential for tumor formation brought on by these aberrant cells can lead to breathing difficulties as well as other health problems. It's a severe condition that frequently calls for medical attention.

Lungs Cancer Often Comes In Two Fundamental **Types**:

I.Non-small Cells Lungs Cancer(NSCLC):It is the most common kind of lung cancer, accounting for about 85% of cases. Some of the subtypes of NSCLC include adenocarcinoma, squamous cell carcinoma, and giant cell carcinoma.

II. Small Cells Lungs Cancer (SCLC):Despite becoming less common, this type spreads and grows more quickly than

NSCLC. It frequently has to do with intensive smoking.

The behavior and outward appearance of the cancer cells under a microscope determine these types of lung cancer. The type of lung cancer affects the treatment options.

Source Or Causes Of Lungs Cancer

I.Tobacco Smoke:The main causes of lung cancer are smoking cigarettes, cigars, and pipes. Tobacco smoke contains harmful compounds that over time harm lung tissue and increase the risk of cancer.

II. Exposure To Radon:A naturally occurring radioactive gas called radon can enter homes through foundational fissures. Long-term exposure to radon at high levels can raise the chance of lung cancer.

III.Air Pollution:Lung cancer risk can be raised by breathing in contaminated air, which may contain dangerous particles and chemicals.

IV.Family History And Genetic Factors:Particularly if there is a history of lung cancer in the family, some people may have a genetic predisposition that makes them more likely to develop the disease.

V.Alcohol Consumption:Lung cancer risk can be increased by heavy alcohol usage, especially if tobacco use is also present.

<u>**Note:**</u>Even if you don't smoke yourself, inhaling smoke from individuals who do can raise your risk of developing lung cancer.

Prevention Of Lungs Cancer.

Adopting a proactive and healthy lifestyle is crucial to lowering your risk of getting lung cancer or any other type of cancer. The following actions can help prevent lung cancer:

I.Quit smoking:The most effective strategy to avoid lung cancer if you smoke is to stop. To help you quit, look for resources and assistance.

Avoid being around people who are smoking, as this poses a serious risk.

II.Avoid Exposure To Harmful Chemical:Reduce your home's and workplace's exposure to asbestos, radon, arsenic, and other toxins.

If you work in locations where exposure to hazardous substances is a possibility, use protective gear and adhere to safety regulations.

III.Healthy Diet And Exercise:Maintain a diet that is well-balanced and full of fresh produce, healthy grains, and lean proteins.

To maintain a healthy weight and general well-being, get frequent exercise.

IV.Reduce Alcohol Consumption:If you do drink, exercise moderation. For instance, men and women should each have no more than two drinks per day.

V.Maintain A Healthy Lifestyle:Aim for a balanced

lifestyle that includes getting enough sleep, managing your stress, and limiting your exposure to contaminants in the environment.

VI.Vaccination:Consider getting the flu shot if you are eligible, and talk to your doctor about getting the pneumococcal vaccine to avoid respiratory infections.

LiverCancer

Hepatocellular carcinoma (HCC), also referred to as liver cancer, is a form of cancer that develops in the cells of the liver. The liver, a crucial organ in the body, is important for the digestion of bile as well as the processing of nutrients and the detoxification of toxic substances.In its early stages, liver cancer may not exhibit any signs and frequently progresses quietly. Chronic hepatitis B or C infections, excessive alcohol use, obesity, diabetes, exposure to specific poisons or chemicals, and specific genetic disorders are all common risk factors for liver cancer.

Abdominal pain, jaundice (a skin and eye yellowing), unexplained weight loss, appetite loss, exhaustion, and swelling in the legs or abdomen are all possible indications of advanced cancer.A liver biopsy is frequently used in the diagnosis process to confirm the presence of cancer cells. Depending on the stage of the disease, a variety of treatments are available for liver cancer, including surgery, liver transplantation, chemotherapy, radiation therapy, targeted therapy, and immunotherapy.For those with liver cancer, a better prognosis and higher overall survival rates depend on early detection and rapid treatment. Early detection and prevention can be aided by routine tests and the management of risk factors.

Hepatocellular carcinoma (HCC), another name for liver cancer, is a form of cancer that originates in the cells of the liver. It can be brought on by a number of conditions, such as chronic liver disease, hepatitis B or C, high alcohol consumption, and obesity. Depending on the kind and stage of the malignancy, treatment options may include surgery, chemotherapy, targeted therapy, immunotherapy, or a liver transplant. For improved results, early detection and treatment are essential.

Early detection and prompt treatment are essential for patients with liver cancer to have a better prognosis and greater overall survival rates. Routine diagnostics and the control of risk factors can help with early detection and prevention.Treatment options may include surgery, chemotherapy, targeted therapy, immunotherapy, or a liver transplant depending on the kind and stage of the cancer. Early detection and treatment are crucial for better outcomes.Fatigue, unexplained weight loss, appetite loss, abdominal pain or tenderness, bloated belly, jaundice (yellowing of the face and eyes), and easy bruising or bleeding are all signs of liver cancer. If you have any unsettling symptoms, it's very important to seek medical advice so they can perform a thorough evaluation.

Causes Of Liver Cancer

Normal liver cells frequently experience DNA alterations that result in uncontrolled proliferation and the formation of tumors. This is how liver cancer typically arises. Several known risk factors can raise the possibility of getting liver cancer, including:

I. Chronic Viral Hepatitis:Hepatitis B virus (HBV) and hepatitis C virus (HCV) infections considerably raise the chance of developing liver cancer.

II. Cirrhosis:persistent alcohol misuse, chronic viral hepatitis, or nonalcoholic fatty liver disease (NAFLD) are common causes of long-term liver injury and scarring.

III. Alcohol abuse:Alcohol abuse that is excessive and continuous raises the risk of developing liver cancer and harms liver cells.

IV. Obesity:Obesity and being overweight can both raise

the chance of developing fatty liver disease and liver cancer.

V. Diabetes:People with diabetes, especially if it is not well controlled, may be more likely to develop liver cancer.

VI. Anabolic steroids use:The risk of liver cancer can increase with prolonged usage of some anabolic steroids.

VII. Aflatoxin exposure: Aflatoxin-contaminated food, which is poisonous material made by specific types of fungi on grains and nuts, can increase the risk of liver cancer.

It's crucial to remember that not everyone who possesses these risk factors will acquire liver cancer; in fact, some people may have the disease even if they don't. A healthy lifestyle, routine medical exams, and screenings can reduce the risk of developing liver cancer. A healthcare expert must be consulted if you have any doubts about your liver's health.

Prevention Of Liver Cancer

Adopting a healthy lifestyle and reducing exposure to risk factors for the disease are two ways to prevent liver cancer. The following are important precautions:

I. Manage diabetes:If you have diabetes, effectively controlling your blood sugar levels by a healthy diet, regular exercise, and taking medications as directed by your doctor will lower your chance of developing liver cancer.

II. Exercise regularly:Regular physical exercise can help you stay in a healthy weight range, improve your general wellbeing, and lower your risk of developing liver cancer.

III. Maintain a healthy weight and diet:Adopt a healthy diet that emphasizes lean proteins, whole grains, and fruits and vegetables. To lower the risk of fatty liver disease and its complications, maintain a healthy weight.

IV. Limit alcohol consumption:In particular, if you have

a history of binge drinking or liver-related issues, limiting or quitting alcohol use can help avoid liver damage and lower the risk of liver cancer.

V. Avoid exposure to toxins and harmful chemicals:Reduce your exposure to substances like vinyl chloride, arsenic, and aflatoxins that are known to raise the chance of developing liver cancer.

Visit your doctor for periodic checkups and screenings on a regular basis to monitor your overall health and catch any potential problems in the early stages.

Keep in mind that controlling and preventing liver cancer effectively depends on early detection and rapid medical action. Consult a healthcare practitioner for specialized

advice and direction if you
have particular questions
regarding the health of your
liver or risk factors.

About the Author

Wilfred Hastings is an American entrepreneur, educator, author of many books and a lecturer.And he's also involved in so many businesses round the country and writing books is one of the best thing in my life.

www.ingramcontent.com/pod-product-compliance
Lightning Source LLC
Chambersburg PA
CBHW070731260726
48660CB00007B/2791